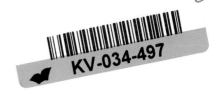
Joint Appointments in Nursing

A Report Prepared for The Commission on Nursing

July 1998

By

PATRICIA LEAHY-WARREN

RGN, RM, Dip. Manag., BSc, H.Dip, PHN.

Public Health Nurse, Southern Health Board
Cork

MARK TYRRELL

RGN, RPN, RNT, BNS, MEd

Lecturer, Department of Nursing Studies
National University of Ireland, Cork

Edited by

DR. GERALDINE McCARTHY-HASLAM

RGN, RNT, MEd, MSN, PhD

Director, Department of Nursing Studies
National University of Ireland, Cork

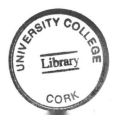

ISBN 0-7076-6130-7

BAILE ÁTHA CLIATH
ARNA FHOILSIÚ AG OIFIG AN tSOLÁTHAIR
Le ceannach díreach ón
OIFIG DHÍOLTA FOILSEACHÁN RIALTAIS,
TEACH SUN ALLIANCE, SRÁID THEACH LAIGHEAN, BAILE ÁTHA CLIATH 2,
nó tríd an bpost ó
FOILSEACHÁIN RIALTAIS, AN RANNÓG POST-TRÁCHTA,
4 - 5 BÓTHAR FHEARCHAIR, BAILE ÁTHA CLIATH 2,
(Teil: 01 - 6613111 — fo-líne 4040/4045; Fax: 01 - 4752760)
nó trí aon díoltóir leabhar.

DUBLIN
PUBLISHED BY THE STATIONERY OFFICE
To be purchased directly from the
GOVERNMENT PUBLICATIONS SALE OFFICE,
SUN ALLIANCE HOUSE, MOLESWORTH STREET, DUBLIN 2,
or by mail order from
GOVERNMENT PUBLICATIONS, POSTAL TRADE SECTION,
4 - 5 HARCOURT ROAD, DUBLIN 2,
(Tel: 01 - 6613111 — ext. 4040/4045; Fax: 01 - 4752760)
or through any bookseller.

£4.00

PREFACE

On March 21st 1997, the Minister for Health, Mr. Michael Noonan, T.D., established the Commission on Nursing. The terms of reference were: to examine and report on the role of nurses in the health service including:

- the evolving role of nurses, reflecting their professional development and the overall management of services;

- promotional opportunities and related difficulties;

- structural and work changes appropriate for the effective and efficient discharge of that role;

- the requirements placed on nurses, both in training and the delivery of services;

- segmentation of the grade;

- training and educational requirements; and

- the role and function of An Bord Altranais generally, including, *inter alia*, education and professional development, regulation and protection of the citizen.

As part of the preparatory work a number of reports were commissioned. This report entitled "Joint Appointments in Nursing" has been prepared by Patricia Leahy-Warren and Mark Tyrrell and edited by Dr. Geraldine McCarthy-Haslam.

Mella Carroll

Ms. Justice Mella Carroll
Chair of the
Commission on Nursing

July 1998

TABLE OF CONTENTS

LIST OF TABLES

INTRODUCTION

The division between nursing practice and education is of major concern to nursing leaders world wide (Elliott, 1997). This gap is deeply entrenched in nursing's past and is well documented in the literature as a historical artefact of nursing's growth and development as a profession (Ford, 1980; Powers, 1976). While it is important to acknowledge the past, it is also incumbent upon contemporary nurses to look to and plan for the future. The survival of nursing as a profession is dependent upon it's ability to develop nursing knowledge in order to ensure improved practice. It is also necessary to monitor and control the domain and quality of practice and the preparation of all nurses. One means of achieving this reunification of nursing lies in the integration of nursing service and education (Ford, 1980).

In this report, Chapter one focuses on the historical evolution of joint appointments in nursing. The diversity of definitions and aims of such appointments are also discussed. This is followed in Chapter two by an analysis of the various existing models of joint appointments. In doing so, the authors identify a number of types of joint appointments, the majority of which were found in the literature from the United Kingdom (UK), the United States (USA) and Canada. The issues of funding and time distribution are presented.

In Chapter three, the scope of joint appointments is evaluated. This entails a review of the literature on role expectations, proposed benefits and limitations of joint appointments. In the final section of this chapter, the writers discuss a number of strategies that can aid the implementation and development of this role. In conclusion a number of pertinent issues relating to joint appointments are raised.

CHAPTER 1

JOINT APPOINTMENTS IN NURSING

1.1 Evolution of Joint Appointments

While joint appointments are a relatively new phenomenon in nursing, the first reference to the concept in the United States dates back to 1929 (Powers, 1976). The author describes an "affiliation agreement" (p. 482) between Yale School of Nursing and New Haven Hospital where a joint education-administration post was established between these two agencies. Powers (1976) is of the opinion that this represented the beginnings of joint appointments in nursing, suggesting that this was very much a far-sighted approach for the time. It would appear however, that the main thrust towards joint appointments in nursing did not occur until the late 1960s and early 1970s, in the United States. Mason and Jinks (1994) suggest that this development came about as a result of the "clinical specialist movement" (p. 1064) that was evident in American nursing at that time. Joint appointments have also featured in the literature from Canada. Wyness and Starzomski (1989) established what they term a "time-exchange joint appointment" (p.35) between the University of British Colombia (UBC) School of Nursing and the Vancouver General Hospital (VGH) Division of Nursing in 1985. However, this joint appointment involved a time-sharing concept of manpower exchange rather than just sharing of financial remuneration.

The first references to joint appointments in nursing in the United Kingdom appear in the literature of the late 1970s and the 1980s (Hewison & Wildman, 1996). In the UK at that time, there was a gradual realisation that something needed to be done about the ever increasing gap between nurse education and practice. This gap had long been acknowledged in the nursing literature of a number of countries, most notably the United Kingdom (Hewison & Wildman, 1996), the United States (Royle and Crooks, 1985), and Canada (Stainton et al., 1989). Such a theory-practice gap, while suggested as early as the latter part of the nineteenth century (Mason & Jinks, 1994), became more evident during the Second World War and reached its peak in the 1970s. The first joint appointment developments in the UK were those at Burford (Wright, 1985, 1984), Oxford (Lathlean and Vaughan, 1994) and at Manchester (Castledine, 1991). Castledine (1991) describes how the first joint appointments in Manchester came about as a result of the first Master's Degree course in clinical nursing. This lead to a combined initiative with Manchester Royal Infirmary whereby a ward sister and charge nurse both worked at the hospital and at the university. The concept of joint appointment arises out of the philosophy of

1

unification, and the belief that nursing education, practice and research should be united (Vaughan, 1990).

1.2 Rationale for Joint Appointments

The rationale for joint appointments can be considered with respect to the theory practice gap and clinical creditbility. Each of these reasons will be addressed in the following paragraphs.

Theory Practice Gap

The theory practice gap has been attributed primarily to the separation of nursing service and education which occurred in North America essentially as a result of the move of nurse education from hospital schools of nursing to university faculties of nursing. The separation of responsibilities was seen to enhance the credibility of nursing education mainly through the establishment of stronger research links (Royle and Crooks, 1985). However, Hewison and Wildman (1996) argue that the move personified "a concrete representation of the distance between education and practice" (p. 754). Pierik (1975) succinctly describes the relationship between service and education when she states:

> Education points an accusing finger at the service and says or implies that they (service personnel) are sincere but are inferior in knowledge to the educators; therefore their patient care (service) is inferior. Service in turn, points an accusing finger at the 'ivory tower' educators and says that while they may know all the 'principles' of patient care, they haven't taken care of a patient for years and are therefore inferior in the area of patient care (Pierik, 1975, p. 567).

Vaughan (1989) maintains that while practice and teaching remain separate in nursing, students will experience a disparity between theory and practice. Joint appointments as evidenced in the literature, have been developed to address the above concerns. Reed and Procter (1993) point to the unequal weighting of value attributed to intellectual knowledge and skills in the general educational system, which results in the clinical skills of nursing being regarded as having lesser status than intellectual abilities. The authors maintain that this distinction is also evident in nursing, a profession which is characterised by a schism' between different types of knowledge of unequal value, namely theory and practice. Thus, whilst theoretical knowledge may have more status, it is perceived by many as being of limited use in the reality of practice. This view is seen as a significant contributory factor to the development of the theory-practice gap. One detrimental effect of the split is that nurse educators are seen as guests when in the clinical setting, (Kramer, 1974).

Taking this a step further, Hutelmyer and Donnelly (1996) assert that the academic culture in the United States shifted from valuing teaching and service to valuing research. Although Universities publicly acclaimed traditions of teaching, service and research at tenure and promotion time, research and publication have reaped the rewards. Clinical practice, often categorised as service, rarely enters the equation for rewards in the academic setting. The authors go on to point out that nurse educators adjusted their scholarship to the demands of the reward system rather than to the core of their discipline, namely, clinical practice (Hutelmyer and Donnelly, 1996).

One attempt to overcome this theory-practice gap was through the Registered Clinical Nurse Teacher, (RCNT), a post which was developed during the 1960's. in the UK. However, it appears from the literature that the clinical teacher role failed because of lack of control over what was taught or practised. This was because the RCNT had little input into curriculum development, did little formal teaching and as a visitor to the clinical areas had no power to influence actual practice or standards of nursing practice (Cave, 1994). In addition, Lathean (1992) in a review of research with RCNT's, showed that clinical teachers were often dissatisfied, mainly due to feelings of low status.

Clinical Credibility

As a result of the demise of the clinical teacher role, the issue of the clinical credibility of those who teach both nursing theory and practice came into question. From the literature it appears that there are different interpretations of clinical credibility. Some authors define it as keeping up to date with current practice, so that what is taught in theory relates to what is carried out in practice (Webster, 1990). Alternatively, clinical competence is defined by Acton et al., (1992) as having expert knowledge of a particular field which can be believed by, and inspire confidence in colleagues and students. It is the opinion of Polifroni and Schmalenberg (1985) that clinical credibility and clinical competence are mandatory if nurse educators are to ensure clinical practice competence of graduates. The authors argue that in order to influence and contribute to the improvement of patient care and nursing care delivery systems, educators must consistently make their presence felt in the clinical arena and earn high credibility among the staff with whom they work. This they claim is also necessary for educators who want to build or test theory through research.

Research conducted in the UK by Crotty (1993) clearly shows that although nurse teachers consider that the clinical teaching of students is important, they should not be expected to perform the function. Furthermore, it is the opinion of Rhead and Strange, (1996), that the historical difficulties in linking theory with practice raises the question for nurse teachers of the importance of educational and clinical credibility. A proposal by Fawcett and McQueen, (1994), was that clinical credibility could be seen in terms of being up to date in theoretical knowledge whilst maintaining some basic skills. In this way, a certain amount of "hands on care" supported by research based knowledge of the current practice would be evident (Crotty, 1993). Another proposal advanced in order to claim clinical credibility, was that teachers should spend a specified number of weeks each year in the clinical practice area to ensure that theoretical teaching was based on current practice. However, it would appear that there is lack of agreement as to whether or not nurse teachers should be required to demonstrate clinical credibility. Some nurse teachers express the view that it is an integral part of their teaching role, while others suggest that they are no longer practitioners and hence should not be required to demonstrate clinical credibility (Jowett et al., 1994).

Cave (1994) stresses that the nursing profession needs to decide exactly the level of clinical ability required to competently teach. In the United Kingdom, a number of models of clinical involvement have been proposed as being appropriate for enabling nurse teachers to maintain their clinical credibility. One such model, that of lecturer-practitioner discussed in section 2.2, has received much attention in the literature (Kirk et al., 1997; Carlisle et al., 1997; Rhead and Strange, 1996; Cave, 1994; Burnard and Chapman, 1990). This concept developed and the role emerged from concern about the difficulties experienced by both practitioners and educators in finding a match between what was being done in practice and what was being taught in theory, as well as a fundamental belief in the value of practice as the origin of much nursing theory.

3

1.3. Definitions of Joint Appointments

There appears to be a lack of agreement in the literature regarding a precise definition of joint appointments in nursing, most definitions referring specifically to the joint appointment of lecturer-practitioner. One example from the UK is that by Fairbrother and Ford (1997). These authors define a lecturer/practitioner as: "someone who is appointed by both a Trust and a university, or who has responsibilities to both a Trust and a university." (p. 32). More specifically, Vaughan (1990) suggests that the lecturer practitioner is someone who has responsibility for both practice and education within a defined clinical area. In Canada , the faculty of nursing at the University of Calgary and the nursing service agencies in Calgary were reported in 1989, to be in the process of establishing a variety of joint appointments with a focus on nursing practice. In this context, a joint appointment refers to a formal agreement of appointment between the faculty of nursing and a nursing service. This was seen to go one step further than the models of appointment that claim a goal of reducing the theory-practice gap. The goal in Calgary was to strengthen congruence between practice, education and research (Stainton et al., 1989). A similar definition from Canada is that by Wyness and Starzomski, (1989) who state that "in a joint appointment a person is employed concurrently by an educational institution and a health care agency, and has responsibilities and priveleges in each" (p. 35). Rokosky, (1979) suggest that joint appointments are derived from an individual educator's interests, and their contacts with a particular agency, or as a response to organisational goals which promote collaboration between nursing practice and education.

Hutelymer and Donnelly (1996) suggest that the involvement of clinicians in educational settings be called reverse joint appointments and where nursing educators are involved in practice be called joint appointments. The overall goal is to bring together education and practice for the purpose of improving conditions of learning , maintaining educator expertise in the clinical area, retaining expert nurses as role models, and incorporating research into practice (Hutelymer and Donnelly, 1996). Powers (1976) emphasises the need for clinical nursing and nursing education to be rationally joined' in order to ensure the progress of both. She argues that a profession is not limited to a body of knowledge, and that it is questionable whether or not there can be significant teaching or research unless it is based on actual nursing practice.

A number of dual appointments are discussed in the literature. While these posts are not necessarily joint appointments in that there is only a single employer involved and there is no sharing of remuneration, they are briefly discussed here as it is felt that they may serve as a model for joint appointments in nursing. Furthermore, the reasons for the establishment of these posts stem from the effort to unify nursing service and nursing education, a goal that is held in common with joint appointments. For example, Turner and Pearson (1989) outline a Faculty Fellowship Programme as one model of uniting nursing service and education. The authors cite Ford and Kitzman's (1983) definition of faculty practice as "those functions performed within a service setting that have as their principal goal the continual advancement of nursing care" (p. 19). This programme involves two distinct components. These include participation as a staff nurse, and engagement in a clinical nursing project. This opportunity is available to all registered nurses who are prepared at Masters' or Doctoral level, and who are employed in a nursing education position during the academic year. Participants in the programme agree to work a minimum of eight weeks during their summer vacation in the clinical setting.

A similar venture is described by Baker et al., (1989), again in the United States. The authors describe a partnership between two unrelated public institutions, the University of South Carolina, and the Richmond Memorial Hospital. The main focus is that the appointee, a unit based clinical nurse specialist, performs a multiplicity of functions including nursing practice, education and research. A third such collaborative appointment is the Adjunct Executive Appointment for Faculty that is described by Kelly et al., (1990). These authors describe a service-education collaboration model based on adjunct executive appointments of nurse educators to health care organisations. This model involves an honorary position at the level just below that of the director of nursing in the nursing services department. The adjunct associate director participates at the department of nursing executive level "with voice but no vote " (p. 37). This appointment was described as without salary. Specific activities varied depending on the agency concerned. Further, while the title provided the opportunity to keep up to date on problems and concerns of practicing nurse administrators, it appears that this position is without autonomy and thus limited in influence (Kelly et al., 1990).

1.4. Aims of Joint Appointments

The aims of joint appointments vary according to the nature of the post, most of those reported in the literature referring to the joint appointment of lecturer-practitioner. Whatever the model, it is generally assumed that such positions will serve to unite theory and practice and promote a unified ideology for all spheres of nursing (Mason & Jinks, 1994). Wright in 1988 for example, suggests that such appointments have one common aim, namely to reduce the gap between theory and practice in nursing. Bond (1985) and Davis (1989) concur with this view, adding that such appointments also help to answer the issue of the clinical credibility of nurse teachers. Tamlyn and Myrick (1995) are more explicit in this regard. These authors state that joint appointments are derived from institutional goals and are usually based on a philosophical agreement that such appointments enhance the development of clinical practice, primarily through nursing research. To this end, the authors argue that recruitment advertisements for such posts often specify requirements that candidates are qualified for the specific joint appointment and emphasise a close university affiliation. This is to ensure that the appointee will maintain a direct link with the university (Tamlyn and Myrick, 1995). One of the aims of joint appointments, identified by Hutelmyer and Donnelly (1996), is to have expert nurse role model the clinical critical thinking so important for nursing practice. Vaughan (1990) suggests that the main aims of the lecturer practitioner are to identify and maintain standards of practice, and prepare and contribute to the educational programme of students in relation to theory and practice of nursing.

Royle and Crooks (1985), in a paper on clinical academic appointments identify a number of goals for post holders. These include: enhancement of the quality of patient care and student learning; contribution to the professional development of both clinical and academic staff and the facilitation of communication between staff from both agencies. Southworth (1992) describes a nursing joint appointment in the UK between public health and District Health Authorities. The main aim of this joint role was to ensure a seamless service that avoided duplication of care provision in the community. Southworth (1992) argues that collaboration at the level of the primary health care team is necessary to ensure that individual's skills are complimentary and not duplicated.

Fairbrother and Ford (1997), in a study of the joint appointment lecturer/practitioner in the Trent region [UK] examined how such posts were established and supported. From the data analysed in this study, the researchers present a number of themes depicting the proposed outcomes of such posts. These include:

- Enhanced relationship between service and education,

- Improved student support,

- Patient-focused practice,

- Increased research skills of post holder,

- Teaching based upon current practice,

- Establishment of good practice areas,

- Trust/Higher Education Institute image raised.

On further analysis, Fairbrother and Ford (1997) identified two recurrent themes, namely, the need for "role clarity," and being "pulled in two directions". Furthermore, it was argued that careful planning is essential for success. In conclusion, the researchers stated that: "Lecturer/practitioners who are aware of the realities of practice are not only appreciated by service and education managers, but also provide the students with excellent role models" (p. 34).

Finally in this regard, Wyness and Starzomski, (1989) point out that the goals of a joint appointment include enhancing the quality of patient care and student learning by fostering an atmosphere of scholarship, inquiry and clinical excellence; contributing to the professional development of both clinical staff and university faculty teaching staff; and fostering communication between members of two organisations.

Summary

While joint appointments are a relatively new phenomenon in nursing, there is evidence in the literature of their exitance dating back to 1929 in the US and to 1970 in the UK. The concept of joint appointments appears to have arisen out of the philosophy of unification, the belief that nursing education, practice and research should be united.The lack of unity, known as the theory practice gap has the potential of becoming greater now than ever, with the worlds of university and clinical nursing further apart than in the past. While the academic culture has encouraged the development of research and other scholarly activities, the literature suggests that this may be to the detriment of clinical practice. The theory practice gap has been further exacerbated by the demise of the clinical teacher role and by the apparent lack of clinical credibility of many nurse educators. Efforts to unify nursing service and nursing education are based on the premise that the professional issues and concerns in nursing can be managed more effectively and efficiently by collaboration between university nursing education departments and nursing service than by either group working in isolation. Joint appointments have been proposed as a logical means of reunifying nursing education and clinical practice.

While there appears to be a lack of agreement in the literature regarding definitions of joint appointments, one common denominator is that they encompass a dual role involving nursing education and clinical practice.

CHAPTER 2

MODELS AND FUNDING IN JOINT APPOINTMENTS

2.1 Models of Joint Appointments in Nursing

Hutelmyer and Donnelly,(1996) have identified two main models for joint appointments, the unification model and the collaboration model. The unification model reflects geographical and administrative unity of the service and education agencies. An example of such a model is that at Rush University, Chicago and the University of Rochester (Ford, 1980), where administration of the clinical agency and the nursing school is unified. Members of the faculty have appointments as both clinicians, and teachers, from the level of Dean (who is also the director of nursing) to that of lecturer/practitioner. This arrangement allows for striving towards a tripartite goal of excellence in nursing practice, education, and research. For example, in 1971, whilst planning for a new school of nursing, it was proposed that nursing service and education be integrated under the leadership of the Dean of nursing, Rochester University. This proposal was based on the belief that such an integration would provide a rational education for students, that it would assist in the upgrading of nursing practice and patient care, and stimulate clinical nursing research (Powers, 1976).

The Collaboration model is an interinstitution model between separate agencies with mutual goals. In this model, the administration of the clinical agency and the school are distinctly separate. Educators have appointments within the hospital and conversely, many nurses in clinical practice hold academic appointments. Furthermore, some of the salary costs may be shared. Examples of these models include developments at Case Western Reserve University USA, and McMaster University, Hamilton, Canada. At Case Western Reserve University joint appointments were established between the University and the University Hospital of Cleveland. In this case the chairman of each clinical major (for example, medical, surgical, paediatric, etc.) for the school of nursing was made responsible for the corresponding clinical speciality within the hospital. This ensured responsibility for both quality patient care and quality nursing education within a single, expert authority. The roles of the dean and nursing administrator were described as giving leadership to each enterprise, collaborating with each other to promote excellent programs of nursing education, clinical practice and research. They were also in the prime positions to procure and allocate essential resources, and give administrative support (Powers, 1976). In the McMaster approach, nurse educators at McMaster University spend the equivalent of a half-day per week in clinical practice. Furthermore, occasionally, this was preceded by a two to four week block of full-time clinical practice (Kergin, 1980).

Within the model of collaboration is the Dyad model, one which involves sharing of services rather than financial exchange. For example at the University of Maryland, educators were paired with clinical nurse specialists in the hospital. Joint projects in education, practice, and research were implemented. Examples of these projects were the establishment of education and support groups for parents in a paediatric unit, and a research project that identified patients at risk for falls and resulted in the development of a falls prevention programme. (Hutelymer and Donnelly, 1996).

According to Royle and Crooks (1985), enshrined in the collaboration model are three types of cross-appointments ; (i) joint appointment: where direct costs are jointly shared by the hospital and the university, (ii) clinical associate appointment, conferred by the hospital to university-funded nursing faculty; and (iii) clinical appointment ; conferred by the university to nursing staff funded by the hospital. In addition, Hutelmyer and Donnelly, (1996) report a fourth model, in which departments of nursing services established the position of the Director of Nursing Research as a joint appointment with a university school of nursing. In this arrangement, the researcher is a faculty member at a university school of nursing with proven ability in conducting nursing research and an interest in developing a research program in a hospital. Simultaneously, the researcher teaches in the school of nursing in the hospital. There is formal agreement between the two institutions regarding specific responsibilities and the percentage of time to be allocated between the nursing department and the school. Salary and benefits are shared between both institutions.

2.2 Types of Joint Appointments

There are various types of joint appointments evident in the literature such as those of advanced practitioner (Castledine 1991a&b), clinical nurse specialist (Menard, 1987), consultant nurses (Wright, 1988), and practitioner-teachers (Vaughan, 1989), the types varying according to the focus of the different aspects of work.

In a review of the literature, Emden (1986) identifies a number of joint appointment types that are commonly used in the UK. The main difference between these posts and those reported from the USA is that these appointments involve the sharing of two jobs by two persons, typically a ward sister/charge nurse and a lecturer in the college of nursing. Ashworth and Castledine (1980) are reported to have held the first of these posts. This joint appointment involved Manchester University and Manchester Area Health Authority. These joint appointees therefore, shared both positions. Salary and conditions were managed by the university and reimbursed by the area health authority. Wright (1983) describes a similar arrangement at Burford, this time involving a clinical nurse teacher post and a charge nurse post. These two posts were shared on a 50:50 basis with another nurse and were jointly remunerated by service and education. Similar approaches to joint appointments and the experiences of those holding them are reported by Burns (1992) and Walden et al., (1982). Davis and Tomney (1982) suggest that there are four elements common within the different types of joint appointments.

These are:

- Agreement between two institutions;
- The appointee is selected by both institutions involved;
- Terms of appointment are negotiated between the appointee and the institutions involved;
- Appointee is an employee of both institutions.

8

Similarly, Arpin (1981) describes three types of joint appointments. These are "status only," whereby a senior member of the nursing service contributes to the university faculty through participation in staff meetings, continuing education courses, student courses, and in some instances may also undertake some teaching. The second type is one whereby the university employs a clinical staff member as a part-time lecturer for 40% of the time. The remaining 60% is directed towards their primary clincial nurse appointment. The third joint appointment described by Arpin (1981) is that of a clinical specialist who is appointed as a clinical associate. The clinical associate is expected to contribute to the overall activity of the faculty and both institutions agree that time must be protected in order not to interfere with the primary role. In addition to acting as a preceptor, the clinical associate is also required to read and comment on students' clinical logs, participate course seminars, and become a member of a thesis committee. This latter type of joint appointment does not seem to accord with those defined elsewhere in the literature. Furthermore, it is not clear who remunerates this post, and at what level. That there is a enormous remit attached to this post is evident from the description above.

Joel (1985) identifies three types of joint appointments in use at Rutgers College of Nursing in the USA. The first type, associate appointees, have a primary appointment with the college, and an associate appointment with the affiliated clinical agency. Appointees are expected to give their time and talent to the hospital, for example through staff inservice development and clinical consultation, or administrative and programme development.

The second type is a clinical appointment, where candidates must hold the credentials appropriate for full faculty status. Appointees are awarded an academic rank commensurate with the educational and experiential background that is specified for such a clinical appointment. Furthermore, they are expected to support the learning of students in the hospital setting and may formally participate in clinical or classroom teaching on an episodic basis. Joel (1985) stresses that the clinical appointment should not be construed as an honourary post, indeed the author argues that their contribution is very much valued.

The third type is the shared appointment. The appointee negotiates the division of time between the two institutions and is primarily employed and remunerated by the school. Polifroni and Schmalenberg (1985) describe another type of joint appointment, that of clinical consultant. These nurses are remunerated jointly by the hospital and the university and work in both places.

Joint appointments are not however the exclusive domain of nurse education. Tamlyn and Myrick (1995) for example suggest that joint appointments should also be offered to nurse administrators and other nurse leaders who can contribute to the area of health-care policy development. Similarly, Southworth (1992) in a paper on the need to decrease the sometimes overlapping roles of the various primary health-care personnel, suggests that joint nursing advice is a crucial element in breaking down boundaries and demarcation lines. This, the author argues, could be achieved by the creation of joint appointments whereby the chief nurse advises both the District Health and Family Health Service Authorities.

2.3 Funding and Time Distribution in Joint Appointments

Tamlyn and Myrick (1994) assert that joint appointments can be either funded or unfunded. Those that are unfunded are generally termed "honorary joint appointments", while those that are funded are termed "joint appointments" (p. 491). According to Royle and Crooks (1985), traditionally, salary differences have existed between clinical and educational institutions. Furthermore, in medicine, doctors who are engaged in education have been remunerated for their joint clinical-academic position. This has not been the case for such posts in the nursing profession. This may be because joint appointments in nursing are a new concept and as such, have not yet been fully evaluated (Royle and Crooks, 1985). Joint appointments according to Wright (1988) are typically held by teachers who are also practitioners. In most cases, they are paid for and managed jointly by the education and service sides of nursing, thus the joint appointee comes under two distinct tiers of nursing organisation. Moreover, Fairbrother and Ford (1997) point out that many of the lecturer-practitioner joint posts in the UK are remunerated outside the Whitley scale salary provisions, this presumably to reflect the experience and qualifications of the post holder.

In one model of joint appointment from the United States, it is reported that each party contributes 50% of the post holders salary (Campbell & King, 1992). The authors identify a number of issues in funding that need to be considered when the contract for this type of joint venture is being prepared. These include publication rights, salaries, evaluation procedures, effective dates, holidays, overtime, vacation times and compensatory times. Another UK example is given in the literature, (Burns, 1992), which identifies how half of the post holders time (and hence half her salary) is spent lecturing at the Oxford Polytechnic, while the other half is spent in clinical and managerial activities in two surgical wards at the John Radcliffe Hospital.

Indeed, many agencies have failed to address the issue of reimbursement policies (Lamont and Cairns, 1989), and where funding arrangements have been established , a variety exist. However, exchange of moneys is a feature of some, but not all joint appointments (Emden, 1986). In some situations apportionment of funds is determined by the amount of time spent in each institution (Elliott, 1997; Hutelmyer and Donnelly, 1996; Wright, 1988; Pierik, 1976). For example, Pierik (1976) describes a shared salary appointment whereby the appointee is a top level clinical nurse who also holds a senior post in education and whose salary is shared accordingly. Similarly, Hutelmyer and Donnelly (1996) describe an arrangement whereby the school of nursing purchases 40% of the joint appointees time, this in order to ensure the involvement of the joint appointee in both clinical teaching, and also in the school's activities. Joel (1985) in describing the experiences of joint appointments at Rutgers College of Nursing, identifies a situation where no moneys were exchanged in the process. Joel (1985) points out that while the institutions could have made an arrangement in this regard, they decided instead to proceed on a negotiated manpower exchange.

It appears that the reason for this decision concerned the time it would have taken to make suitable financial arrangements. In this instance, joint appointees contribute 20, 25, 33 or 40 per cent of their effort and hence their time to the institution of secondary appointment (the college), however, they continue to receive a salary and benefits from the hospital. In a recent conjoint appointment in Australia, Elliott (1997) outlined how the appointee provided two days each per week both to the University as lecturer and to the hospital as a middle manager (Assistant Director of Nursing) with no direct-line responsibilities, but with a focus as a researcher of management issues. The fifth day was used as flexi-time to be used by the appointee as necessary. A formal contract was signed by the three parties and issues such as benefits and entitlements, salary etc. were negotiated. However, the appointee was directly responsible to both the Head of Department and the Director of Nursing respectively, for institution-specific matters.

Other examples of joint appointments where salary and time are negotiated are also reported in the literature (Wright, 1988; Menard, 1987). Emden (1986), in a review of a joint college (40%), hospital (60%) arrangement at the Royal Adelaide Hospital, Australia, demonstrates how "it was agreed the college would reimburse the hospital at intervals throughout the year for the appropriate portion of the joint appointee's regular salary" (p. 31). However, it is not always the case that the partner who pays the majority of the funding receives the greater portion of the joint appointees time. For example, in Georgetown University, Washington, Lachat et al., (1992) report how the joint appointee splits responsibilities between the Department of Nursing (75%), and the School of Nursing (25%). While the position was funded by the hospital, the college offered "reciprocal consultation, research assistance, committee membership and lecture expertise" (p. 56), to the School of Nursing.

Summary

A number of models of joint appointments have been identified in the literature and these are broadly categorised as unification, collaboration and dyad models. Within these models are a number of types of joint appointments, the most common of which in the UK is the lecturer-practitioner. In North America, the term "faculty practice" is commonly used to describe a plethora of education/clinical joint roles. Where funding arrangements have been established, a variety of schemes have been pursued ranging from complete funding from one of the parties, to shared funding based on time distribution. However, it must be borne in mind that exchange of moneys is a feature of some but not all joint appointments.

CHAPTER 3

THE SCOPE OF JOINT APPOINTMENTS IN NURSING

3.1   Roles and Responsibilities of Joint Appointees

The nature of joint appointments, the format they take and the roles and responsibilities of the joint appointee, vary according to the needs of the specific situation. Indeed, Joel (1985) argues that the role requirements of the joint appointee appear extreme because of the constant shift from one working world to the other. Moreover, the roles and responsibilities of the joint appointee are very much determined by the constituent posts involved. For instance, Black et al., (1989) in a paper on the experiences of nursing joint appointments in a Teaching Health Unit in Ontario, Canada, highlight the roles of the appointees from the service perspective. While the project concerned joint appointees from a number of disciplines including nursing, medicine and epidemiology, the paper concentrated on a description of the clinical projects carried out by nursing joint appointees. These included:

- Self-medication practices for the elderly;

- Nursing theories: models and frameworks for practice;

- Development of critical appraisal learning packages;

- Immigrant health promotion project.

While the roles and responsibilities were specific to each project, the projects shared a number of similar characteristics in accordance with the objectives of the Teaching Health Unit. These were:

- Encourage collaboration among students, managers and staff;

- Influence the structure and function of service delivery;

- Provide impetus for the development, funding and dissemination of community health research;

- Improve knowledge and skills of staff and students about current critical/ community health issues (Black et al., 1989).

Royle and Crooks (1985) argue that the cultural milieu of both the hospital and the academic institution differ considerably and hence have different expectations regarding the roles and responsibilities of the joint appointee. In essence, the joint appointee requires a sense of professional autonomy and ability to generate their own rewards to enable them to survive within these diverse cultures. The scope of the joint appointee's responsibilities according to Royle and Crooks (1985), requires that appointees are highly qualified, competent practitioners who possess a well defined philosophy of nursing and teaching expertise. MacPhail (1975) expresses the view that joint appointees need to be risk takers, and willing to try new approaches and assume responsibility for nursing practice, education and research. This view correlates with that expressed by Wright (1991) who argues that joint appointees must demonstrate excellence in practice if they are to uphold the values and expectations of the role.

Joel (1985) identifies a number of responsibilities of the various types of joint appointees at Rutgers University College of Nursing, as outlined in Table 3.1 below:

TABLE 3.1.   Joint Appointee Responsibilities

Appointment type	Responsibilities
Associate Appointment	Enhance nursing care; provide quality nursing practice for the students.
Clinical Appointment	Support the activities of students within the hospital; to act as a role model for students.
Shared Appointment	Providing leadership in developing programmes for nursing care, education and research.

Source: **Joel, L. (1985) The Rutgers Experience.** *Nursing Outlook.* **33 (5): 222.**

It would appear from the above table that the associate and clinical appointments broadly equate to a mentorship/preceptorship role. The shared appointment has similar attributes to a joint appointment in that it incorporates clinical, research and educational components.

The activities of clinical consultant joint appointees generally fall into six categories. These are outlined by Polifroni and Schmalenberg (1985) as: direct patient care; role modelling; in-service education; projects; information resource; head nurse support. The authors indicate that the functions of clinical consultants differ depending on the particular clinical area, it's circumstances and needs. Therefore, a precise job description was not created, rather the appointee was allowed to determine most of the parameters of the role.

Fairbrother and Ford (1997) set out two main areas of responsibility for the lecturer-practitioner, the most popular type of joint appointment in the United Kingdom. These are the identification and maintenance of standards of nursing policies and practice in clinical areas, and the teaching of nursing theory and practice. According to these authors, the title "lecturer/practitioner" implies a dual role, namely that of lecturing and practising. Hence the authors argue, in order for the post holder to be effective in these roles, they must possess both academic and clinical credibility.

Vaughan (1989) suggests that the joint appointment role is one of "unification" whereby the responsibilities for teaching, practice, management and research are vested in one person. Thus the author points out, the lecturer-practitioner manages a clinical unit, establishes the policies and styles of work organisation, is responsible for staff development and has autonomy in regard to the budget and staff skill mix. Vaughan further asserts that the joint appointee "has responsibility for teaching both the theory and practice of nursing within the clinical setting. Furthermore, alongside other nurse teachers, the lecturer-practitioner will have input to the overall curriculum design." (Vaughan, 1990, p.52).

According to Mason and Jinks, (1994), Vaughan's model was based on the premise that the practitioner-teacher would replace the ward sister and would have responsibility and authority for both nursing practice, management and education in a defined clinical area. The strength of the role is the potential to enhance the relationship between service and education. An important factor is the joint appointees contribution to curriculum planning, thus ensuring it is grounded in the real world of practice (Fairbrother and Ford, 1997). Finally in this regard, Woodrow, (1994) argues that even when the role has been defined, successors to a previously established post should develop their own role and remain dynamic by responding to changing needs.

3.2 Proposed Benefits of Joint Appointments

A plethora of benefits have been attributed to joint appointments in nursing. Wright (1988) for example suggests that the assumption is that the teacher of nursing when in charge of the ward will produce a climate conducive to educational and practical ideals. According to the author, students should be able to learn and give nursing care, and attrition rates should be reduced through student empowerment. Mason and Jinks (1994) see the joint appointees role as a significant improvement on the traditional clinical teachers, however, Vaughan (1990) points out that the latter had no authority in clinical areas and only a limited role in educational settings. Conversely, the joint appointee holds defined clinical responsibilities and is therefore in a position to influence the practice of nursing. Indeed, it has been suggested that the answer to the dual problems of clinical credibility of nurse teachers, and the theory practice divide can only be found by joint appointments (Fawcett & McQueen, 1994). This view is supported by a number of other authors including Fairbrother and Ford, (1997); Hewison and Wildman, (1996); Cave (1994); Emden, (1986); Wright, (1985). According to Elliott (1997), most nurse practitioners are unable to manage simultaneously the service, education, consultation, and research component of their professional role which often results in fragmentation and frustration. The author argues however that a joint appointment is a method of achieving practice in all of the above areas, while bridging any perceived gap between the service and education institutions (Elliott, 1997).

A further proposed benefit of joint appointments is that identified by Ingram (1994), who suggests that experienced practitioners have a need to occupy a role within which theory can be both generated and taught. The author argues that by having a formalised role within these two areas, the nurse can allow for each to inform the other, thus aiding the diffusion of all of Carper's (1978) four forms of knowledge in clinical practice. Fairbrother and Ford, (1997) warns however, that if the lecturer-practitioner initiative is to succeed, purchasers will need to be convinced of the value of such posts. Therefore, the post holder will have to be able to demonstrate the value brought to practice and education settings. To this end, joint appointees must evaluate, research and publish their work (Castledine, 1991).

Benefits of joint appointments reported by university staff include an increase in self confidence, a more realistic teaching approach, an enhancement in the quality of care (Arpin, 1981), and the opportunity to meet the professional expectations for practice, education and research (Royle and Crooks, 1985). Other benefits of joint appointments recounted in the literature concerned individual professional development (Wright,1988; Walden et al., 1982), enhanced theory and practice for students (Elliott, 1997; Hutelmyer and Donnelly,1996) and improved communication and co-operation between institutions (Rasmussen, 1984). Despite the issues of role strain and ambiguity (discussed below), the benefits of these posts appear to outweigh the costs (Wright, 1991).

While the benefits of joint appointments for improved student learning and for enhancement of patient care are evident in the literature, there is little consideration given to the role that joint appointees could play in influencing policy at the hospital or at governmental levels (Acorn, 1987; Davis and Tomney, 1982; Arpin, 1981; MacPhail, 1975). Some further benefits to the role of the joint appointee are outlined in Appendix I.

3.3   Limitations to the Role of Joint Appointments

Despite their many successes, a number of limitations and difficulties with joint appointment posts are reported in the literature. According to Elliott (1997), the majority of joint appointments include a hospital role with functions such as ward/unit manager, as well as a teaching role. The result of combining these two complex roles is that the joint appointee inevitably experiences varying degrees of ambiguity and role strain. Consequently, the joint appointee frequently juggles two "full-time" positions (Rasmussen 1984). Wright (1988) himself one of the earlier proponents of joint appointments of the lecturer-practitioner type, identifies role conflict, stress, burnout and work overload as some of the potential problems associated with such roles. Similarly, Fairbrother and Ford (1997) report that joint appointees find themselves stretched to such an extent by the competing requirements of university life that supporting students in practice is difficult. The authors further suggest that lecturer-practitioners in particular are required to meet the competing demands from colleagues in practice and education which can result in their being pulled in opposite directions.

Rhead and Strange (1996) argue that the expectation of fulfilling two roles places on the joint appointee the double imposition of developing and maintaining two roles at a credible level. Indeed, Arpin (1981), states that while there are many benefits of joint clinical-educational appointments, appointees report that that there was insufficient time to develop either role to their satisfaction. This was primarily due to their being torn apart between two positions with different demands.

Wright (1988) describes how in many instances the demands of these posts were too great and as a result few posts remain in their original form. However, some of the principles have been incorporated into the more recently developed lecturer practitioner roles. Work overload is central to the arguments on limitations made by a number of other authors including Vaughan, (1989), and Lamont and Cairns, (1989). One comparative study however, found no differences in role ambiguity between joint appointees and traditional faculty (Acorn, 1991). This author concludes from a study of five Canadian University nursing faculties with the largest proportion of joint appointees (n = 113), that assuming a joint appointment does not necessarily mean that the post holder will experience an increased level of role conflict and role ambiguity. The author further suggests that joint appointees do not differ from traditional nurse educators in levels of role conflict and role ambiguity, scholarly productivity levels, or job satisfaction. Acorn (1989) also found that role conflict was more prevalent than role ambiguity, and was buffered by the presence of social support.

Mason and Jinks (1994) in a review of the literature on the role of the practitioner-teacher in nursing, identify a number of disadvantages of such roles. These include:

- Two roles are superimposed with little consideration of which parts of each role can be discarded (Vaughan, 1990).

- The joint appointee is sometimes considered to be too inexperienced for the teaching part of the role (Powers, 1976).

- The position is not easily graded or incorporated into existing structures (Pearson, 1983).

- Because the joint appointment encompasses two organisations, the appointee is subject to both role and interpersonal conflict (Wright, 1988).

The cultural diversity of the respective partners in joint appointments has already been mentioned. This has also been identified a source of difficulty for the joint appointee. For example, Hutelmyer and Donnelly, (1996) comment that "the difference between the two cultures can be a major source of dissonance for the joint appointee" (p. 74). These authors point out that the ethos of service differs very much from that of education. Nursing service values quality patient care, and therefore, little time is devoted to conduct and supervise research and other scholarly activities. Conversely, the educational system emphasises knowledge development both for the individual and for the profession. This situation is often compounded by the fact that the appointee is not always an experienced educator nor someone who is familiar with the universities expectations of it's academic staff (Lachat et al., 1992), this as a result of their not having experienced university education themselves (French, 1992).

The relationship of the joint appointee to management is also identified as a potential area of conflict. Woodrow (1994a) suggests that lecturer-practitioners whose roles are ambiguous, may become management led. The author further argues that in such a case there is a risk that the lecturer-practitioner will become just another "pair of hands" to ease the workload. This has also been identified by Emden, (1986) as a limitation to the post. Woodrow (1994a) further argues that budgetary pressures may tempt some managers to dispense with lecturer-practitioners who appear to provide poor value for money. Other writers warn that joint appointees may have to divide their loyalties between clinical nursing and education, rather that seeking common ground between them (Davis, 1989; Vaughan, 1989). These authors conclude that the divisions within nursing which traditionally have prevented it's professional growth and independence are still perpetuated despite the development of joint appointments.

Moreover, Vaughan (1989) concludes that "while the sentiment behind the concept of joint appointee is admirable, this role needs some kind of superman or woman to do the job properly." (p.52). The author further commenting from the perspective of someone who has held such a post states: "it is almost impossible to do the job well" (p. 52). Clearly, some of these difficulties could have been avoided with better planning and/or better management support (Wright, 1988). Some further limitations to the role of the joint appointee are outlined in Appendix I.

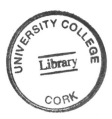

3.4. Facilitating and Supporting the Role of the Joint Appointee in Nursing

Joel (1985) suggests that the key to success with joint appointments lies in "protecting the pioneers who accept shared appointments from themselves and from the system" (p.223). If left unsupported, joint appointees tend to see their role as encompassing two full-time jobs. Furthermore, the requirement that appointees acquire a masters or doctoral degree and engage in scholarly activity as well as clinical teaching, may create overload. Hence, the appointee must be well supported and protected (Joel, 1985). Administrative support is vital for the success of joint appointments (Wyness and Starzmoski, 1989). Similarly, Royle and Crooks (1985) suggest that joint roles should be planned in conjunction with nursing administration. The authors argue that the administrator is a valuable resource person who can facilitate integration into and across organisational lines and structures. Acorn, (1989), in the previously mentioned study, suggests that support from administration and peers can alleviate the dysfunctional effects of role conflict. It is therefore incumbent on administrators to clarify the expectations of joint appointees and monitor the presence of conflict and ambiguity to prevent dysfunctional levels (Acorn, 1989).

Campbell and King (1992) acknowledge a number of characteristics of the public health administration-academic joint appointee that are necessary in order to "maintain sanity"(p. 26). These include appointees being excellent time managers, efficient secretarial support system, ability to delegate responsibility and to maintain a sense of humour, and a realisation that "they could not do all things for all people at all times" (p. 26). Similarly, Royle and Crooks, (1985) indicate the importance of open communication, mutual support and flexibility in the joint appointee, nursing service managers, and in nurse academics. The authors further outline a number of other strategies for implementation and maintenance of joint clinical-academic appointments in nursing, and as set out in Table 3.2.

TABLE 3.2. **Strategies for implementation and maintenance of joint clinical-academic appointments in nursing**

---

1. Goal-directed, mutually planned entry.
2. Administrative support.
3. Open communication.
4. Promotion of professional autonomy.
5. Peer support.
6. Willingness to take risks.
7. Clinical and educational expertise.

Source: **Royle and Crooks, (1985): Strategies for Joint Appointments.** *International Nursing Review.* **32 (6): 187.**

Other necessary supports are identified by Lamont and Cairns, (1989). These include release time from current duties, altered schedules, sabbaticals, leaves of absence without pay, and other financial remuneration. The authors further support the assertion that the greatest facilitator of faculty practice is administrative support.

According to Vaughan (1990), in order to facilitate the development of the role of joint appointee, the first step is to make available more free time in the role of the current ward sister/charge nurse role. This the author suggests can be brought about in two ways. First of all, a system of primary nursing needs to be introduced and thus, many of the traditional ward sister tasks will be shed. Secondly, the introduction of staff support roles which provide a service to practitioners, will mean that many of the hassles in the day to day life of the senior nurse can be lightened. Finally, the introduction of secretarial support at clinical level could take over some of the administrative tasks. The purpose behind all these changes according to Vaughan (1990), is to free time for other work. Similarly, Wright, (1988) identifies the essential elements of support as being commitment, skills and preparation of the joint appointee, and co-ordination through one designated manager agreed by both service and education. This the author believes will lead to commitment and support from education department managers, and from service managers and colleagues. Despite the problems associated with such posts, Wright (1988) hastens to say that where the above criteria have been met, many joint appointees have prospered to the benefit of students, patients, the organisation and themselves.

Finally, Elliott (1997), on evaluating a conjoint appointment involving a nursing management role, makes a number of recommendations in this regard. These were that the appointees' teaching commitment should be less than half of the total full-time equivalent teaching hours; that the appointment should be made at a level that will accord the appointee sufficient authority to enable them to function autonomously at all levels of both institutions and that the appointment will acknowledge the need for ongoing and continual education of the appointee.

Summary

It appears from the literature reviewed that the nature of joint appointments, the format they take and the roles and responsibilities of the joint appointee varies according to the needs of the specific situation. In the UK, the roles and responsibilities of the lecturer-practitioner have been identified as the establishment and maintenance of standards of nursing care, and the teaching of nursing theory and practice in the clinical areas. Similar responsibilities are identified from the North America literature. Issues such as the enhancement of nursing care, the provision of quality nursing practice for students, and the support of students in the clinical areas, are considered fundamental. However, it must be stressed that for post holders to be effective in their roles, the possession of both academic and clinical credibility is essential. A plethora of benefits have been attributed to joint appointments. These primarily relate to the appointee, the student and the institutions involved. Personal benefits reported include an increase in self confidence, a more realistic teaching approach, satisfaction due to an enhancement of the quality of care. Chief among the benefits for the student were exposure to an expert role model with ability to relate theory to practice in a coherent way. Reported benefits to the institutions concern an increase in quality patient care due to the application of nursing research to clinical practice. Conversely, a number of limitations have also been attributed to joint appointments, including work overload, unrealistic expectations, and poor understanding of joint appointments.

The literature also suggests it is essential that joint appointees are carefully chosen, with respect to academic achievements and personal characteristics. The key to a successful joint appointment is believed to lie in supporting the joint appointee, ensuring that the appointment is at a senior level, and according them adequate autonomy.

CONCLUSION

The concept of joint appointments in nursing are a relatively recent phenomenon, and appear to have arisen out of the philosophy of unification. This philosophy emerged from the concern that a disparity existed between what was taught in the classroom and what occurred in practice. This theory – practice gap has been further exacerbated by the move of nurse education into the higher education setting, and also by the demise of the clinical teacher role. University culture values academic activities more so than clinical practice, and hence many nurse educators in pursuing academic excellence have failed to maintain clinical credibility.

It is argued by some authors that one of the more effective and efficient means of unifying nursing service and education is by joint appointments. This is based on the premise that such appointments require collaboration between nursing service and education. A multitude of benefits of joint appointments are extolled in the literature and these are given further credence by the fact that many of the authors concerned were themselves joint appointees. These benefits accrue not only to the appointee and the student, but also to the establishments concerned. Paramount among these benefits is the development of nursing research, it's application to clinical practice, and the fostering of an atmosphere of scholarship, inquiry and clinical excellence. Consequently, this contributes to the professional development of both clinical staff and university faculty, and the enhancement of communication between members of both organisations.

Despite the foregoing, a number of limitations of joint appointments have been identified. These primarily concern role operationalisation, and problem areas include role strain due to work overload and unrealistic expectations, and role ambiguity due to poor understanding of joint appointments. Indeed, in many cases the two composite roles of the joint appointment have been merged with little or no thought given to aspects of either role which could have been discarded. While a number of models and types of joint appointments have been identified in the literature, the classification systems which are commonly used to describe these are sometimes confusing. Compounding this is the lack of agreement regarding definitions of joint appointments. One consequence of this is that it is difficult to make comparisons between the various authors' accounts. It is evident from the literature that there is no overall agreement with regard to how these posts are funded, or how time is distributed, and hence little guidance in these regards is available to those planning to embark on such an endeavour.

A number of strategies to maintain and support joint appointees are identified in the literature. Serious consideration should be given to issues such as selection of candidates, the level of appointment necessary to function autonomously, mutual agreement on roles and responsibilities, conditions of tenure and employment, and support structures such as office accommodation and secretarial assistance. Management from both organisations must also be cognisant of their differing cultural perspectives. Failure to acknowledge this may lead to the premature departure of the appointee from the post. Conversely, implementation of the position is facilitated when managers provide support and freedom for the joint appointee to move within two independent systems. Mutual awareness of goals on the part of management and staff of both institutions help promote communication and an understanding of the roles and scope of practice of the joint appointee.

While it is evident from the literature reviewed in this project that there is much to commend joint appointments, the writers strongly recommend that those planning to embark on such an initiative ensure that the necessary structures are in place prior to initiating such an appointment. Factors influencing the functioning of joint appointees have been identified and strategies to facilitate functioning presented. The joint appointee must be accorded independence in thought and action, yet be capable of working within the boundaries of two social systems with differing values and expectations. Those concerned can provide the supports necessary to overcome the barriers identified and to achieve the rewards inherent in successful implementation of what is clearly an exciting and innovative role.

REFERENCES

Acton, L., Gough, P. and McCormack, B. (1992) The clinical nurse tutor debate. *Nursing Times* 88 (32), 38-41.

Arpin, K. (1981) Joint appointments: strengthening the clinical practice component in nursing education programmes. *Nursing Papers* 13 (2), 9-14.

Ashworth, P. and Castledine, G. (1980) A joint service educational appointments in nursing. *Medical Teacher* 2 (6), 295-299.

Baker, M., Boyd, N.J., Stasiowski, S.A. and Simons, B.J. (1989) Interinstitutional collaboration for nursing excellence: Part 1. Creating the partnership. *JONA* 19(2), 8-12.

Black, M., Edwards, N., McKinght, J., Valaitis, R. and VanDover, L. (1989) Experiences of nurse joint appointments in a teaching health unit. *Public Health Nursing* 63, 135-140.

Bond, S. (1985) Part of the union. *Senior Nurse* 2 (4), 12-13.

Burnard, P. and Chapman, C. (1990) Nurse Education: The Way Forward. London: Scutari Press.

Burns, S. (1992) Grading practice. *Nursing Times* 88 (1), 40-42.

Campbell, B. and King, J. (1992) Public health service administration and academia. *Journal of Nursing Administration* 22 (12), 23-27.

Carlisle, C., Kirk, S. and Luker, K. (1997) The changes in the role of the nurse teacher following the formation of links with higher education. *Journal of Advanced Nursing* 24, 762-770.

Carper, B. (1978) Fundamental patterns of knowing in nursing. *Advances in Nursing Science* 1 (1), 13-23.

Castledine, G. (1991a) The advanced nurse practitioner: Part 1. *Nursing Standard* 5 (43), 34-36.

Castledine, G. (1991b) The advanced nurse practitioner: Part 2. *Nursing Standard* 5 (44), 33-35.

Cave, I. (1994) Nurse teachers in higher education- without clinnical competence, do they have a future? *Nurse Education Today* 14, 394-399.

Crotty, M. (1993) Clinical role activities of nurse teachers in Project 2000 programmes. *Journal of Advanced Nursing* 18 (4), 460-464.

Davis, J. (1989) Who or what are LPs? *Senior Nurse* 9 (10), 22.

Davis, L. and Tomney, P. (1982) The best of two worlds: An appraising look at joint appointments in Canada today. *Canadian Nurse* 78 (8), 34-37.

Elliott, D. (1997) A conjoint appointment involving a nursing research management role. *International Journal of Nursing Practice* 3, 47-52.

Emden, C. (1986) Joint appointment: An Australian study illuminates world views. *The Australian Journal of Advanced Nursing* 3 (4), 30-41.

Fairbrother, P. and Forde, S. (1997) It's a duet, not a duel. *Nursing Times* 93 (16), 31-34.

Fawcett, T.N. and McQueen, A. (1993) Clinical credibility and the role of the nurse teacher. *Nurse Education Today* 14, 264-271.

Ford, L.C. and Kitzman, H.J. (1983) Organisational perspectives on faculty practice: Issues and challenges, in Barnard, K.E. (Ed) *Structure to Outcome: Making it work*. Paper presented at the first annual symposium on nursing faculty practice. American Academy of Nursing.

Ford, L.C. (1980) Unification of nursing practice, education and research. *International Nursing Review* 27 (6), 178-183, 192.

French, S. (1992) Reform in higher education for nurses: comparative comments from Canada. *Contemporary Nurse* 1 (2), 54-67.

Hewison, A. and Wildman, S. (1996) The theory-practice gap in nursing: a new dimension. *Journal of Advanced Nursing* 24, 754-761.

Hutelmyer, C. and Donnelly, G. (1996) Joint appointments in practice positions. *Nursing Administration Quarterly* 20 (4), 71-79.

Joel, L. (1985) The Rutgers experience: one perspective on service-education collaboration. *Nursing Outlook* 33 (5), 220-224.

Jowett, S., Walton, I. and Payne, S. (1994) *Challenges and Change in Nurse Education. A Study of the Implementation of Project 2000*. Slough: National Foundation for Educational Research.

Kelly, K., Gardner, D. and Johnson, M. (1990) Adjunct executive appointment for faculty: an innovation in nursing collaboration. *Journal of Nursing Administration* 20 (10), 35-42.

Kirk, S., Carlisle, C. and Luker, K. (1997) The implications of Project 2000 and the formation of links with higher education for the professional and academic needs of nurse teachers in the United Kingdom. *Journal of Advanced Nursing* 26, 1036-1044.

Kramer, M (1974) *Reality Shock*. St. Louis: Mosby.

Lachat, M., Zerbe, M. and Scott, C. (1992) A new clinical educator role. *Journal of Nursing Staff Development* March/April, 55-59.

Lamont, P. and Cairns, B. (1989) Nursing faculty and clinical practice. *The Canadian Nurse* September, 22-25.

Lathlean, J. and Vaughan, B. (Eds) (1994) *Unifying Nursing Practice and Theory*. Oxford: Butterworth Heinemann.

Lathlean, J. (1992) The contribution of lecturer-practitioners to theory and practice in nursing. *Journal of Clinical Nursing* 1, 237-242.

MacPhail, J. (1975) Promoting collaboration between education and service. *The Canadian Nurse* May, 32-34.

Mason, G. and Jinks, A. (1994) Examining the role of the practitioner-teacher in nursing. *British Journal of Nursing* 3 (20), 1063-1072.

Menard, S. (1987) Possibilities and Predictions, in Menard, S. (Ed) *The Clinical Nurse Specialist: Perspectives on Practice*. New York: John Wiley and Sons, 213-226.

Pearson, A.(1983) *The Clinical Nursing Unit*. London: Heinemann.

Pierik, M. (1975) Joint appointments: collaboration for better patient care. *Nursing Outlook* 21 (9), 576-579.

Polifroni, E.C. and Schmalenberg, C. (1985) Faculty practice that works: two examples. *Nursing Outlook* 33 (5), 226-228.

Powers, M.J. (1976) The Unification Model in Nursing. *Nursing Outlook* 24 (8), 482-487.

Rasmussen, D. (1984) Joint appointments: a staff nurses view. *Journal of Nurse Education* 23 (6), 267-269.

Reed, J. and Procter, S. (1993) Nursing Knowledge: A Critical Examination, in Reed, J. and Procter, S. (Eds) *Nurse Education: A Reflective Approach*. London: Edward Arnold.

Rhead, M. and Strange, F. (1996) Nursing lecturer-practitioners: can lecturer-practitioners be music to our ears? *Journal of Advanced Nursing* 24, 1265-1272.

Royle, J. and Crooks, D. (1985) Strategies for joint appointments. *International Nursing Review* 32 (6), 185-188.

Southworth, A. (1992) A seamless service for community care. *Nursing Standard* 6 (27), 40.

Stainton, M., Rankin, J. and Calkin, J. (1989) The development of a practicing nursing faculty. *Journal of Advanced Nursing* 14, 20-26.

Tamlyn, D. and Myrick, F. (1995) Joint nursing appointments: a vehicle for influencing health care change. *Journal of Advanced Nursing* 22, 490-493.

Turner, D.M. and Pearson, L.M. (1989) The faculty fellowship programme: uniting service and education. *JONA* 19 (10), 18-22.

Vaughan, B. (1990) Knowing that and knowing how: the role of the lecturer-practitioner, in Kershaw, B. and Salvage, J. (Eds). *Models of Nursing*. London: Scutari Press.

Vaughan, B. (1989) Two roles- one job. *Nursing Times* 85 (11), 52.

Walden, E., Sander, R. and Gallant, K. (1982) Sharing the pleasure and the pain. *Nursing Times* 78 (20), 833-836.

Webster, R. (1990) The role of the nurse teacher. *Senior Nurse* 10 (6), 21-22.

Woodrow, P. (1994a) Role of the lecturer practitioner: 1. *British Journal of Nursing* 3 (11), 571-575.

Woodrow, P. (1994b) Role of the lecturer practitioner: 2. *British Journal of Nursing* 3 (12), 611-614.

Wright, S. (1991) The nurse as a consultant. *Nursing Standard* 5 (20), 31-34.

Wright, S. (1988) Joint Appointments: Handle with care. *Nursing Times* 84 (1), 32-33.

Wright, S. (1985) Reflecting on Joint appointments. *Senior Nurse* 3 (6), 8-9.

Wright, S. (1984) A climate for learning. *Senior Nurse* 1 (20), 20-21.

Wright, S. (1983) Joint appointments. The best of both worlds? *Nursing Times* 79 (42), 25-29.

Wyness, A. and Starzomski, R. (1989) Joint appointments revisited. *Canadian Nurse* September, 35-37.

APPENDIX

ADVANTAGES AND DISADVANTAGES
OF JOINT ACADEMIC/CLINICAL APPOINTMENTS

Advantages	Disadvantages
EDUCATORS	
—job satisfaction	—heavier workload
—respect from students and staff	—role strain/burnout
—maintain clinical competence and skills	—increased energy & time demands
—research opportunities	—no recognition for tenure/promotion
—control over learning situations	—division of responsibilities
—decreased preparation time for classes in clinical area	—lack of focus while in the clinical area
—may provide additional income	
STUDENTS	
—exposure to demonstrated expert practice	—sense faculty role confusion
—availability of good learning experiences	—loss of consulting due to faculty dual responsibilities
—direct involvement with future employers	
NURSING RELATIONSHIP	
—communication between service and education	—agency/service availability and co-operation
—sharing of resources e.g.: guest speakers	—resentment of non-practising – faculty related to lack of participation in committees
—mutual identification of needs for research	—unclear lines of responsibility
—mutual understanding of objectives and problems	
—increase visibility of nurse practitioners to the community	
CLIENTS	
—high quality of patient care	—interruptions in continuity of care

Adapted from: **Lamont, P. and Cairns, B. (1989) Nursing Faculty and Clinical Practice** *The Canadian Nurse* **September, 22-25.**

Wt. P60015. 500. 9/98. Cahill. (M29156). G. Spl.